HASHIMOTO'S ENCEPHALOPATHY MANAGEMENT DIET COOKBOOK

Nourishing Recipes For Cognitive Wellness:

Healing Meals For Brain Health-

Delicious Dishes For Neurological Support

DR. SHAYLA LEWIS

Table of Contents

DISCLAIMER

Write a brief complete Disclaimer for my diet cook book telling them that the author is not in any association with any company, business or individual and also this book is written by the authors knowledge and understanding

The information provided in this diet cookbook is based on the author's personal knowledge and understanding. The author is not affiliated with, endorsed by, or associated with any company, business, or individual. The recipes and dietary advice contained within this book are intended for informational purposes only. Readers should consult with a healthcare professional or a registered dietitian before making any significant changes to their diet or lifestyle. The author assumes no responsibility for any adverse effects that may result from the use or misuse of the information contained in this book.

CHAPTER ONE
Understanding Hashimoto's Encephalopathy

Hashimoto's Encephalopathy (HE) is a rare autoimmune condition that causes brain inflammation as a result of antibodies attacking healthy tissue. While it is named after Hashimoto's thyroiditis, an autoimmune thyroid illness, the two are not the same thing.

HE symptoms can range from cognitive impairment to confusion, seizures, stroke-like events, hallucinations, tremors, and coma. Because these symptoms can mirror other neurological diseases, identifying HE can be difficult. However, early detection and treatment are critical for controlling the disease and avoiding long-term consequences.

HE can have a substantial influence on daily living, making previously normal chores more difficult. Memory issues, difficulties concentrating, and exhaustion can all hurt jobs, social activities, and relationships. Additionally, the unpredictability of symptoms can cause dissatisfaction and anxiety.

Importance of Nutrition

Nutrition is essential for controlling Hashimoto's Encephalopathy and encouraging recovery. A well-balanced diet can assist to reduce inflammation, promote brain function, and improve general well-being. Because HE is an autoimmune disorder, specific dietary changes may help relieve symptoms and boost the immune system.

Choosing nutrient-dense foods high in antioxidants, vitamins, and minerals can help minimize oxidative stress and inflammation in the brain. Consuming foods high in omega-3 fatty acids, such as fatty fish, flaxseeds, and walnuts, may also have anti-inflammatory properties. Maintaining steady blood sugar levels with a healthy diet can also help prevent energy dumps and improve cognitive performance.

The fundamentals of low-carb, antioxidant-rich, and anti-inflammatory diets.

Low-carb, antioxidant-rich, and anti-inflammatory diets are frequently recommended for treating autoimmune diseases such as Hashimoto's Encephalopathy. These dietary practices are intended to reduce inflammation, improve immunological function, and boost overall health.

A low-carb diet focuses on consuming less carbs, particularly refined sweets and grains, which can promote blood sugar increases and inflammation. Instead, it focuses on natural meals like vegetables, fruits, lean protein, and healthy fats.

An antioxidant-rich diet comprises a variety of fruits, vegetables, nuts, seeds, and herbs that contain chemicals that help to battle oxidative stress and inflammation. Berries, leafy greens, colorful vegetables, and herbs like turmeric and ginger are particularly high in antioxidants.

An anti-inflammatory diet aims to reduce substances that can cause inflammation, such as processed meals, refined carbohydrates, trans fats, and excessive alcohol. Instead, it promotes full, nutrient-dense foods with anti-inflammatory characteristics, such as fatty fish, olive oil, nuts, seeds, and spices.

Getting started with cooking

Getting started in the kitchen might be intimidating for new cooks, but it doesn't have to be. Begin with easy recipes that need a few materials and equipment. Look for recipes that fit your dietary needs and constraints, and don't be afraid to experiment with flavors and ingredients.

Purchase basic kitchen tools and equipment, including a nice chef's knife, cutting board, pots, and pans, and measuring cups and spoons. Learn basic cooking techniques such as chopping, sautéing, roasting, and boiling, then gradually develop your talents as you gain confidence in the kitchen.

Meal planning can also help to expedite the cooking process and ensure that you have nutritious meals available when you need them. Make a grocery list before going to the supermarket to minimize impulse purchases and stay within your budget. Consider batch cooking and meal planning on weekends to save time during the busy week.

Building a Support System

Managing a chronic ailment such as Hashimoto's Encephalopathy can be difficult, but having a strong support system can be quite beneficial. Surround yourself with compassionate friends, family members, healthcare practitioners, and online groups that can provide encouragement, advice, and emotional support.

Joining Hashimoto's Encephalopathy support groups or online forums can help you feel more at ease and connected. Sharing your experiences, coping tactics, and resources with others who understand what you're going through can be quite beneficial.

If you're having difficulty dealing with the emotional toll of living with a chronic ailment, don't be afraid to seek professional help. Therapy, counseling, and support groups designed expressly for people with chronic illnesses can help them develop coping skills and provide emotional support. Remember that you are not alone, and there are people and services available to assist you deal with the difficulties of living with Hashimoto's Encephalopathy.

CHAPTER TWO

Introduction to Low-Carb Diets: Hashimoto's Encephalopathy (HE) is an uncommon autoimmune condition that causes brain inflammation. While the specific reason is unknown, controlling symptoms frequently entails dietary changes to reduce inflammation and promote overall well-being. In this chapter, we look at the advantages of following a low-carb diet as part of HE treatment.

Reducing carbohydrate intake can have several beneficial impacts on HE symptoms. For starters, it helps to stabilize blood sugar levels, preventing energy troughs and emotional swings that are commonly associated with HE. Carbohydrates, particularly processed carbohydrates, can cause blood sugar increases followed by sharp reductions, and worsening symptoms such as weariness and cognitive impairment. Individuals with HE can maintain more steady energy levels throughout the day by eating low-carb foods.

Furthermore, a low-carb diet may lower inflammation throughout the body, including the brain, which is critical for treating HE symptoms. Carbohydrates, particularly those abundant in sweets and processed grains, can cause inflammation, exacerbating the neurological symptoms of HE. Individuals with HE who eat complete, nutrient-dense foods low in carbs may be able to reduce some of the inflammatory burden on their bodies, resulting in enhanced cognitive performance and overall well-being.

Low-Carb Meal Planning: When planning meals on a low-carb diet, careful consideration is required to guarantee appropriate nutrition while staying within target carbohydrate intake levels. Here are some suggestions for incorporating low-carb meals into everyday menus for those with Hashimoto's Encephalopathy:

Emphasise Whole Foods: Build your meals around non-starchy veggies, lean proteins, healthy fats, and small servings of low-glycemic fruits. These foods supply necessary nutrients while limiting carbohydrate intake.

When it comes to carbohydrates, choose complex sources like quinoa, sweet potatoes, and legumes, which deliver fiber and nutrients without producing dramatic blood sugar increases.

Mindful Portion Control: Pay attention to portion proportions, especially while eating carbohydrate-rich foods. Even healthful foods, such as fruits and whole grains, can contribute to carb intake if ingested in significant quantities.

Experiment with Substitutions: Look into low-carb alternatives to standard high-carb foods. Cauliflower rice and zucchini noodles, for example, can be used to replace grains in recipes such as stir-fries and spaghetti, lowering overall carbohydrate intake.

organize Ahead: Make the effort to organize your meals and snacks ahead of time to ensure that low-carb options are always available. This can help prevent impulsive decisions that could undermine nutritional goals.

Individuals with HE can use these meal-planning strategies to prepare nutritious, delicious meals that meet their health objectives while effectively managing symptoms.

Delicious Low-Carb Recipes: In this section, we've compiled a list of simple recipes that are low in carbohydrates but full of flavor. These recipes are not only delicious but they are also designed to help people manage Hashimoto's Encephalopathy. From robust salads to savory main courses, each meal is designed to deliver nourishment while keeping carbohydrate intake under control.

Some examples of low-carb recipes are: Grilled chicken Caesar salad with homemade dressing.

Cauliflower crust pizza topped with fresh vegetables.

Zucchini noodles with pesto and cherry tomatoes.

Baked salmon with lemon and dill.

Turkey lettuce wraps with avocado and spicy mayonnaise.

These recipes demonstrate the variety of low-carb ingredients and prove that cutting carbs does not entail compromising flavor or satisfaction. Individuals with HE can enjoy a variety of foods while efficiently controlling their symptoms by integrating these delectable recipes into their meal plans.

Snacking Smartly: Snacking can be a trap for those on a low-carb diet, but with proper planning, it can be an opportunity to fuel the body and quell cravings. Here are some nutritious low-carb snack alternatives to help people with Hashimoto's encephalopathy remain on track:

Nuts and Seeds: A handful of almonds, walnuts, or pumpkin seeds has protein, healthy fats, and fiber, making it a filling and nutritious snack.

Vegetable Sticks with Dip: Crunchy veggies like carrots, celery, and bell peppers mixed with hummus or guacamole provide a delightful low-carb snack high in vitamins and minerals.

Plain Greek yogurt sprinkled with fresh berries is a creamy and tasty snack high in protein and antioxidants. Choose full-fat yogurt to keep carbs low.

Hard-boiled eggs are a handy, quick, and high-protein snack that is ideal for satisfying hunger between meals.

Cheese and Deli Meat Roll-Ups: Wrap slices of deli meat around cheese sticks or avocado slices for a quick and filling snack that is low in carbs but great in flavor.

Individuals with HE can maintain steady energy levels and minimize blood sugar changes throughout the day by eating nutrient-dense, low-carb snacks.

Dining Out Strategies: Eating out can be difficult for people on a low-carb diet, but with some help, it is feasible to navigate restaurant menus while adhering to dietary guidelines. Here are some tips for eating out while controlling Hashimoto's Encephalopathy:

Review Menus in Advance: Many restaurants now offer online menus, allowing customers to compare alternatives and plan ahead. Look for foods that are inherently low in carbohydrates or can be readily adapted to meet your nutritional requirements.

Choose Protein-Based recipes: Look for recipes that feature lean proteins such as grilled chicken, fish, or steak. These selections are often lower in carbohydrates and can be used with non-starchy veggies to provide a balanced meal.

Ask for Substitutions: Don't be afraid to request substitutions or modifications to accommodate your low-carb diet. Request more veggies instead of rice or potatoes, or a salad instead of bread on the side.

Be Wary of Hidden Carbs: Sauces, dressings, and condiments may contain hidden carbohydrates. Ask for sauces on the side or questions about the ingredients to ensure they meet your dietary needs.

Portion Control: Restaurant portions are frequently greater than necessary, so divide a meal with a dining buddy or ask for a half portion to avoid overindulging.

Individuals with HE can enjoy meals at restaurants while adhering to their dietary objectives if they use these dining tactics. They may maintain a low-carb lifestyle while enjoying dining out by making informed decisions and advocating for their needs.

CHAPTER THREE

Understanding antioxidants:

Antioxidants are chemicals that play an important function in lowering oxidative stress in the body. Oxidative stress occurs when the body's free radicals and antioxidants are out of balance, causing damage to cells, proteins, and DNA. In the setting of Hashimoto's Encephalopathy (HE), reducing oxidative stress is critical because it can aggravate inflammation and worsen symptoms.

Explaining how antioxidants reduce inflammation and promote brain function is critical. Antioxidants operate by neutralizing free radicals, which are unstable chemicals that can damage cells and contribute to inflammation. Antioxidants, by scavenging these free radicals, aid in reducing inflammation and protect against oxidative damage, promoting general brain health.

In the treatment of Hashimoto's Encephalopathy, integrating antioxidants into the diet is critical to battle inflammation and oxidative stress, potentially relieving symptoms and increasing general well-being.

Incorporating antioxidant-rich foods:

Including a variety of fruits, vegetables, nuts, seeds, whole grains, and herbs in your diet is an excellent approach to guarantee you get enough antioxidants. Fruits high in antioxidants include berries (blueberries, strawberries, raspberries), citrus fruits (oranges, lemons, limes), and tropical fruits (pineapple, papaya).

Leafy greens (spinach, kale, Swiss chard), cruciferous vegetables (broccoli, cauliflower, Brussels sprouts), and colorful vegetables (bell peppers, tomatoes, carrots) are all high in antioxidants, including vitamins A, C, and E, as well as phytonutrients.

Simple strategies for incorporating antioxidant-rich foods into meals include adding berries to muesli or yogurt for breakfast, serving a colorful salad for lunch, snacking on nuts and seeds, and incorporating a variety of vegetables into soups, stews, and stir-fries for dinner.

Antioxidant-Rich Recipes:
Mouthwatering dishes with antioxidant-rich components can help manage Hashimoto's Encephalopathy symptoms. Examples include:

Make a Berry Blast Smoothie with mixed berries (strawberries, blueberries, raspberries), spinach, Greek yogurt, almond milk, and protein powder for a nutritious breakfast or snack.

For a tasty and nutritious lunch, combine cooked quinoa with roasted vegetables (e.g., red peppers, cherry tomatoes, zucchini, and red onion), fresh herbs (e.g., parsley and basil), lemon juice, olive oil, and feta cheese.

For a delicious and antioxidant-rich main course, grill or bake salmon fillets and top with a homemade salsa of berries, red onion, jalapeño, cilantro, lime juice, and honey.

Superfood Spotlight:

Highlighting antioxidant-rich items can provide insight into crucial elements to include in the diet to manage Hashimoto's Encephalopathy. Some notable superfoods with high antioxidant content are:

Berries, including blueberries, strawberries, raspberries, and blackberries, include antioxidants such as anthocyanins, vitamin C, and flavonoids that can reduce inflammation and prevent oxidative stress.

Leafy greens, like spinach, kale, Swiss chard, and collard greens, include antioxidants like vitamin C, E, and beta-carotene that promote brain function and reduce inflammation.

Almonds, walnuts, chia seeds, and flaxseeds include antioxidants such as vitamin E, selenium, and polyphenols, which promote brain function and minimize oxidative stress.

Meal Prep Made Easy:
Including antioxidant-rich foods in meal planning and preparation can be made easier with these practical tips:

Plan your week's meals ahead of time, including antioxidant-rich options.

Prepare ingredients ahead of time to save time during hectic weekdays.

Prepare large batches of antioxidant-rich dishes, like soups, stews, and casseroles, to freeze for subsequent meals.

Use shortcuts such as pre-cut vegetables, frozen berries, and canned beans to save time and maintain nutrition.

Individuals suffering from Hashimoto's Encephalopathy can improve their brain health, reduce inflammation, and effectively manage symptoms by following these measures.

CHAPTER FOUR

Accepting Anti-Inflammatory Eating

Hashimoto's Encephalopathy (HE) treatment frequently requires a multimodal approach, with dietary changes playing an important part. Chapter 4 of the "Hashimoto's Encephalopathy Management Diet Cookbook" dives into the fundamentals of an anti-inflammatory diet, explaining how it can help people with HE reduce symptoms and improve their general well-being.

The role of inflammation:

Inflammation plays a critical role in the pathophysiology of Hashimoto's Encephalopathy, worsening neurological symptoms and decreasing cognitive function. Understanding how inflammation affects the brain and body is critical in developing appropriate management techniques. In HE, the autoimmune response attacks the thyroid gland, causing the secretion of proinflammatory cytokines and the activation of immune cells. These inflammatory mediators can cross the blood-brain barrier, causing neuroinflammation and contributing to the typical neurological symptoms of HE, such as disorientation, seizures, and psychosis.

Furthermore, chronic inflammation triggers a chain reaction of negative consequences on general health, raising the risk of comorbidities like cardiovascular disease, diabetes, and neurological illnesses. Individuals with HE who treat inflammation through dietary changes may be able to reduce immunological dysregulation, relieve neurological symptoms, and improve their quality of life.

Anti-inflammatory Foods to Include:

The chapter includes extensive recommendations for anti-inflammatory foods that can be used as the foundation of a therapeutic diet for those with HE. The cookbook promotes a plant-centric approach that nourishes the body and reduces inflammation by focusing on nutrient-dense whole foods high in antioxidants, omega-3 fatty acids, and phytonutrients. The key components of an anti-inflammatory diet are:

Fruits and veggies: Colourful fruits and vegetables are high in vitamins, minerals, and antioxidants, which fight oxidative stress and reduce inflammation. Incorporating a variety of produce, such as berries, leafy greens, cruciferous vegetables, and citrus fruits, ensures a wide range of phytonutrients with strong anti-inflammatory qualities.

Cold-water fish such as salmon, mackerel, and sardines contain high levels of omega-3 fatty acids, which are known for their anti-inflammatory properties. Furthermore, flaxseeds, chia seeds, and walnuts are plant-based providers of these important fats, which regulate immunological function and reduce inflammatory responses in the body.

Whole grains: Fiber-rich whole grains including quinoa, brown rice, and oats reduce inflammation by stabilizing blood sugar levels and improving gastrointestinal health. Unlike refined grains, which promote inflammation, whole grains give long-lasting energy and promote metabolic balance.

Healthy fats: Consuming monounsaturated and polyunsaturated fats, such as avocados, olive oil, and almonds, reduces inflammation and improves brain function. These heart-healthy fats act as building blocks for cell membranes and aid in the absorption of fat-soluble vitamins, promoting overall health.

Flavorful anti-inflammatory recipes:

To demonstrate the practical use of anti-inflammatory food principles, the cookbook includes a variety of delectable meals that will tantalize the taste senses while nurturing the body. From vivid salads overflowing with fresh vegetables to rich soups loaded with aromatic herbs and spices, each recipe prioritizes anti-inflammatory components while maintaining flavor. Examples of tasty anti-inflammatory foods include:

Turmeric-seasoned lentil soup with kale and coconut milk.

Grilled salmon and citrus-herb quinoa salad.

Roasted veggie medley with balsamic glaze and fresh herbs.

berry-almond smoothie bowl topped with hemp seeds and granola.

These exquisite recipes not only fulfill culinary appetites but also act as powerful allies in the fight against inflammation, providing a pleasant way to promote healing and vitality.

Mindfulness Eating Practices:

In addition to fueling the body with anti-inflammatory foods, mindful eating habits promote a comprehensive approach to symptom management in HE. Mindfulness requires paying attention to body cues, enjoying each meal, and cultivating a nonjudgmental awareness of the eating experience. Individuals with HE who practice mindfulness during meals can improve digestion, reduce stress-related inflammation, and build a stronger relationship with food and its healing potential.

Here are some techniques for adding mindfulness to mealtime:

Engaging the senses: Pay attention to the colors, textures, and scents of food, increasing sensory awareness and cultivating appreciation for the culinary experience.

Eating slowly and savoring each meal entails chewing deliberately, pausing between bites to savor the flavors and textures of food, and allowing satiety signals to register.

Cultivating thankfulness entails expressing gratitude for the nutrients offered by food while understanding the effort and resources necessary in its preparation.

Portion control: Pay attention to hunger and fullness cues, and eat until satiated rather than indulging mindlessly.

Individuals with HE can cultivate a harmonious relationship with food by incorporating mindfulness into mealtime routines, resulting in increased enjoyment, contentment, and symptom relief.

Maintaining the benefits of anti-inflammatory food necessitates long-term lifestyle changes that prioritize health and wellness. The chapter offers techniques for adopting anti-inflammatory practices into daily life, allowing people with HE to make informed decisions that help them on their journey to wellness. Key considerations include:

Meal planning and preparation: Develop a repertoire of anti-inflammatory recipes and create a meal planning routine to ensure that nutrient-dense meals are always available. Batch cooking and meal preparation might help you stay on track with your diet.

Creating a supportive environment: Surround yourself with a network of family and friends who understand and respect your eating habits. Create a healthy eating environment in your house, complete with nourishing products and culinary utensils to help you prepare meals.

Seeking expert advice: Speak with a qualified dietitian or healthcare physician who understands autoimmune disorders and nutritional treatments. Collaborate to create a personalized nutrition plan based on your specific needs and preferences, with regular follow-ups to track success and make adjustments as needed.

Embracing holistic wellness practices: Combine anti-inflammatory food with stress-reduction tactics, regular physical activity, enough sleep, and other lifestyle changes that improve overall health and resilience. Prioritise self-care and develop habits that nourish the body, mind, and spirit, promoting a balanced and long-term approach to well-being.

Individuals with HE can cultivate resilience, improve health outcomes, and regain control of their health journey by embracing long-term lifestyle changes based on anti-inflammatory principles.

In conclusion, Chapter 4 of the "Hashimoto's Encephalopathy Management Diet Cookbook" provides a complete guide on adopting an anti-inflammatory diet as a cornerstone of HE treatment. The chapter empowers people with HE to harness the healing potential of nutrition and cultivate a vibrant, thriving life by explaining the role of inflammation, providing practical recommendations for anti-inflammatory foods, showcasing flavorful recipes, advocating mindful eating practices, and outlining strategies for long-term lifestyle changes.

CHAPTER FIVE

Understanding Diabetes: Examining the link between Hashimoto's Encephalopathy and diabetes.

Hashimoto's Encephalopathy (HE) and diabetes are two separate medical illnesses, however, they can coexist in some people, creating severe health management issues. Understanding the relationship between these two situations is critical for effectively controlling them.

Hashimoto's Encephalopathy is an autoimmune illness that causes brain inflammation as a result of antibodies attacking healthy brain tissues. While the actual origin of HE is unknown, it is thought to be associated with autoimmune thyroid illness, notably Hashimoto's thyroiditis. This disorder primarily affects the thyroid gland, resulting in hypothyroidism, but it can also cause neurological symptoms like seizures, confusion, and cognitive impairment in certain cases.

Diabetes, on the other hand, is a metabolic condition characterized by elevated blood sugar levels caused by either insufficient insulin production (Type 1) or the body's inability to efficiently use insulin (Type 2). Uncontrolled diabetes can cause a variety of issues, including cardiovascular disease, nerve damage, and kidney problems.

Hashimoto's Encephalopathy and diabetes share an autoimmune component. Both illnesses include immune system dysregulation, which causes inflammation and tissue damage throughout the body. While HE predominantly affects the brain and thyroid, diabetes targets the pancreas and insulin control processes.

Individuals with Hashimoto's Encephalopathy may be at a higher risk of acquiring diabetes, especially if they also have autoimmune thyroid disease. Similarly, patients with diabetes may be more susceptible to autoimmune disorders such as HE due to underlying immune system malfunction.

Managing both illnesses necessitates a comprehensive approach that addresses their own issues while taking into account their interactions. Close symptom monitoring, regular medical check-ups, and adherence to treatment protocols are critical for improving health outcomes in those who have Hashimoto's Encephalopathy and diabetes.

Blood Sugar Management: Tips for monitoring blood sugar levels and making dietary adjustments as needed.

Blood sugar control is crucial for diabetics to avoid complications and preserve good health. Because Hashimoto's Encephalopathy can impair neurological function and cognitive capacities, effectively managing blood sugar levels becomes even more important to avoid increasing neurological symptoms.

Diabetes management relies heavily on regular blood sugar monitoring. This usually entails using a glucose meter to measure blood sugar levels at several points during the day, such as before and after meals, and then modifying insulin or medicine doses accordingly. Individuals with Hashimoto's Encephalopathy should seek support from carers or healthcare experts while managing this aspect of their health, particularly if cognitive impairment is present.

Diabetes patients' blood sugar levels are heavily influenced by their diet. A well-balanced diet rich in whole foods, complex carbohydrates, lean proteins, and healthy fats will help manage blood sugar levels and offer necessary nutrients for overall health. In the case of Hashimoto's Encephalopathy, dietary considerations may include items that promote brain health and cognitive function, such as omega-3 fatty acids found in fish, nuts, and seeds.

Carbohydrate intake is especially crucial for those with diabetes since carbohydrates have the greatest impact on blood sugar levels. Carbohydrate counting is a strategy for estimating the number of carbs in food and adjusting insulin doses accordingly. This includes learning how to read food labels, measure portion sizes, and monitor carbohydrate intake throughout the day.

In addition to carbohydrate counting, meal timing, and distribution can influence blood sugar levels. Eating smaller, more often meals can help to reduce blood sugar rises and crashes, while also providing a consistent source of energy for the body and brain. Individuals with Hashimoto's Encephalopathy and diabetes should consult with a qualified dietitian or healthcare professional to create a personalized meal plan that fits their nutritional needs while also supporting blood sugar management and cognitive function.

Diabetic-Friendly meals: Delicious meals designed to satisfy the needs of people with diabetes.

With the correct recipes and supplies, you can prepare delicious and nutritious meals that help with blood sugar management. Diabetic-friendly meals have fewer added sugars, processed carbohydrates, and bad fats while including lots of fiber-rich foods, lean proteins, and healthy fats.

When creating diabetic-friendly recipes for people with Hashimoto's Encephalopathy, it is critical to consider not just blood sugar control but also cognitive performance and overall brain health. Ingredients high in antioxidants, vitamins, and minerals can aid improve cognitive performance and reduce inflammation in the brain.

Here are some crucial elements to remember while developing diabetic-friendly dishes for people with Hashimoto's Encephalopathy:

Choose whole, unprocessed foods over refined grains like white bread and pasta. Examples include quinoa, brown rice, and oats. Include a variety of fruits and vegetables that are high in fiber, vitamins, and minerals.

Choose healthy fats: Eat avocado, nuts, seeds, and olive oil, and minimize saturated and trans fats found in fried foods, processed snacks, and fatty cuts of meat.

Pay attention to portion sizes: Portion control is critical for blood sugar management and keeping a healthy weight. Use measuring cups, spoons, or a food scale to get exact portion sizes.

Limit the use of added sugars in recipes by substituting natural sweeteners such as stevia, monk fruit, or fruit purees for refined sugar. Be aware of hidden sugar sources in processed foods and beverages.

Experiment with herbs and spices: Instead of seasoning with salt or sugar, use herbs and spices to enhance the flavor of your dishes. Herbs such as basil, cilantro, and rosemary can enhance the flavor and complexity of meals without adding calories or carbohydrates.

Individuals with Hashimoto's Encephalopathy and diabetes can enjoy a broad variety of delicious and nutritious meals that promote their overall health and well-being by adhering to these rules and becoming creative in the kitchen.

Carbohydrate Counting Made Simple: Methods for determining carbohydrate intake and controlling insulin levels.

Carbohydrate counting is a useful method for diabetics to manage their blood sugar levels efficiently. Understanding how different foods affect blood sugar and learning to calculate carbohydrate consumption allows people to make informed dietary choices and alter insulin dosages as needed to maintain optimal blood sugar management.

For people with Hashimoto's Encephalopathy who also have diabetes, carbohydrate counting can be very helpful in supporting cognitive function and minimizing blood sugar fluctuations that can exacerbate neurological symptoms.

Here are several ways to make carbohydrate counting simple and manageable:

Learn to recognize carbohydrate-rich foods: Carbohydrates can be found in a variety of foods, including grains, starchy vegetables, fruits, dairy products, and sweets. Carbohydrate counting begins with learning to recognize these items and estimate their carbohydrate quantity.

CHAPTER SIX

 Food labels contain important information regarding the carbohydrate content of processed foods. When reading labels, keep in mind the portion size and total carbohydrates per serving. When food labels are unavailable, reference materials and smartphone apps can be used to determine the carbohydrate content.

Accurately measuring portion sizes is critical for determining carbohydrate intake. Use measuring cups, spoons, or a food scale to correctly portion foods and track carbohydrate intake.

Keep a food diary: Keeping a food journal will help you track your carbohydrate intake and discover blood sugar patterns. Keep track of your meals, snacks, portion sizes, and blood sugar readings to better understand how different foods affect your blood sugar.

Consult a certified dietitian: A registered dietitian can offer personalized carbohydrate counting and meal planning advice based on an individual's dietary needs, health goals, and medical history. They may assist you in developing a carbohydrate counting plan that is tailored to your dietary tastes and lifestyle while also supporting your overall health and well-being.

Individuals with Hashimoto's Encephalopathy and diabetes can control their blood sugar levels, and improve cognitive function, and general health by learning the fundamentals of carbohydrate counting and adopting these tactics into their daily lives.

Managing Hashimoto's Encephalopathy with diabetes can be difficult, but patients do not have to face these problems alone. Individuals and carers can access a variety of resources and support networks for information, assistance, and emotional support.

Here are some recommended resources and support networks for people dealing with both Hashimoto's Encephalopathy and diabetes:

Establishing a collaborative connection with healthcare providers such as endocrinologists, neurologists, primary care physicians, and registered dietitians is critical for the management of both disorders. These specialists can provide personalized information, treatment recommendations, and continuing support based on individual needs.

Patient advocacy organizations: The American Diabetes Association (ADA), the Thyroid Foundation of America, and the Brain

Foundation offer valuable resources, educational materials, and support services to people suffering from diabetes, thyroid disorders, and neurological conditions such as Hashimoto's Encephalopathy. These organizations frequently provide online forums, support groups, and educational events where people may interact with others suffering from similar issues and share their experiences and advice.

Social media platforms and online forums can be useful sources of support and information for people dealing with Hashimoto's Encephalopathy and diabetes. Joining online forums dedicated to these disorders allows people to interact with peers, ask questions, share tips and strategies, and receive encouragement and understanding from others who are going through similar experiences.

Books, websites, podcasts, and other educational tools can provide useful information for managing Hashimoto's Encephalopathy with diabetes. Look for sites that provide practical advice, evidence-based information, and personal experiences from people who have successfully managed these disorders.

Local support groups for people with diabetes and autoimmune disorders can offer possibilities for connection, information, and emotional support. These groups, which can meet in person or digitally, provide a secure environment for people to discuss their experiences, concerns, and successes with others who understand what they're going through.

Individuals with Hashimoto's Encephalopathy and diabetes can enhance their quality of life by utilizing these services and support networks.

Navigating Neuropathy

Understanding Neuropathy: Neuropathy is defined as damage or dysfunction of one or more nerves, which often results in numbness, tingling, weakness, or pain, particularly in the hands and feet. Neuropathy may coexist with Hashimoto's Encephalopathy due to the condition's autoimmune nature. The immune system's attack on the thyroid gland can cause inflammation, which affects nerves throughout the body. Understanding this relationship is critical for successfully managing both illnesses.

The Hashimoto's Encephalopathy Management Diet Cookbook emphasizes the need to recognize and treat neuropathy symptoms in addition to managing

Hashimoto's Encephalopathy. Individuals can take proactive actions to reduce the impact of neuropathy on their everyday lives by knowing how it presents and how it is related to the underlying autoimmune condition.

Lifestyle changes have an important part in managing neuropathy symptoms. This involves eating a well-balanced diet, exercising regularly, and making other lifestyle modifications that promote nerve health. The cookbook includes practical suggestions for introducing neuropathy-friendly foods into regular meals, such as those high in vitamins B12, B6, and E, which are required for nerve function.

Exercise is also emphasized as an important aspect of neuropathy care. Walking, swimming, and yoga can help to increase circulation, reduce inflammation, and relieve symptoms. Additionally, stress management practices such as meditation and deep breathing can supplement dietary changes and exercise in boosting general nerve health.

Neuropathy-Friendly Recipes: **The cookbook contains a selection of nutrient-dense recipes meant to promote nerve health and ease neuropathy symptoms. These recipes emphasize the use of key nutrients such as antioxidants, vitamins, and minerals that have been shown to improve nerve function.**

Neuropathy-friendly meals include dishes that feature:

Omega-3 fatty acids are present in fatty fish such as salmon, almonds, and seeds.

Vitamin B12-rich foods include lean meats, dairy products, and fortified cereals.

Antioxidant-rich fruits and vegetables include berries, spinach, and kale.

Magnesium-rich foods include legumes, whole grains, and leafy greens.

Individuals who follow these recipes can fill their bodies with the nutrients required to maintain nerve health while eating great and pleasant meals.

Mind-Body activities: In addition to dietary changes and exercise, mind-body activities are promoted as effective aids for controlling neuropathy symptoms. Mindfulness meditation, progressive muscle relaxation, and guided imagery are all techniques that can aid with stress reduction, relaxation, and neuropathic pain relief.

The cookbook explains how to incorporate these practices into your everyday routines, including basic exercises and recommendations for beginners. Individuals with neuropathy symptoms can improve their general well-being and quality of life by embracing mind-body activities in addition to other lifestyle changes.

Seeking Professional Guidance: While lifestyle changes can help manage neuropathy symptoms, it is critical to seek professional advice for personalized management options. Healthcare professionals, such as physicians, neurologists, and dietitians, can make personalized suggestions based on a patient's unique needs and medical history.

The cookbook recommends that users consult with healthcare specialists to establish thorough neuropathy management plans. Depending on the severity and underlying causes of neuropathy, treatment may include pharmaceutical management, physical therapy, or specialized nutritional therapies.

Individuals who collaborate with healthcare practitioners can obtain the assistance and information they require to properly manage neuropathy symptoms and enhance their overall quality of life while living with Hashimoto's Encephalopathy.

CHAPTER SEVEN
Meal Planning and Preparation

Hashimoto's Encephalopathy Management Diet Cookbook offers detailed assistance not just on recognizing the problem but also on how to properly manage it through dietary changes. Chapter 7 looks into the critical component of meal planning and preparation, emphasizing its importance in simplifying dietary management and lowering stress for people living with Hashimoto's Encephalopathy (HE).

Importance of Meal Planning

Meal planning is an essential tool for people with HE since it provides a systematic method for addressing dietary demands. Individuals who plan meals ahead of time can guarantee that they achieve their nutritional needs while sticking to the dietary restrictions imposed by their disease. This proactive strategy eliminates the ambiguity surrounding mealtime decisions and lowers the possibility of accidentally consuming trigger foods that worsen symptoms.

Furthermore, meal planning allows people to take control of their nutrition, which fosters a sense of autonomy and self-efficacy in controlling their health. It enables improved treatment of symptoms such as fatigue and cognitive impairment by providing stable energy levels throughout the day via well-balanced meals.

Create a Meal Plan:

Developing a balanced and satisfying meal plan entails many critical elements that are adapted to the specific dietary requirements of people with HE. The cookbook offers step-by-step instructions to make this procedure easier, taking into account nutrient requirements, food allergies, and individual tastes.

First, people are urged to analyze their dietary needs depending on age, gender, activity level, and any comorbidities. This serves as the foundation for defining meal composition, ensuring that appropriate nutrients are provided to maintain general health and manage HE symptoms.

Then, clients are assisted through the process of identifying appropriate food sources that meet their dietary requirements.

This may entail avoiding frequent trigger foods like gluten, dairy, and processed sweets while focusing on nutrient-dense options high in vitamins, minerals, and antioxidants.

Efficient grocery shopping is vital for keeping a well-stocked kitchen that meets dietary needs and tastes. The cookbook's smart purchasing tactics help people traverse grocery aisles with confidence, making informed selections that fit into their meal plan.

Key advice includes making a grocery list based on scheduled meals to avoid impulse purchases and waste, carefully reading product labels to discover potential allergens or hidden substances, and choosing fresh, whole foods whenever feasible. Individuals are also advised to visit alternate shopping locations, such as farmers' markets or specialty health food stores, to gain access to a greater variety of healthful ingredients.

Time-saving Meal Preparation Tips:

Incorporating time-saving meal prep techniques into the weekly routine can considerably reduce the burden of cooking, particularly during hectic times. The cookbook provides practical tips for streamlining meal preparation, allowing people to eat healthful cooked meals without sacrificing valuable time and energy.

Batch-cooking core foods like grains, beans, and meats to have on hand for easy meals throughout the week is one example of a time-saving meal prep strategy. Preparing veggies ahead of time by cleaning, cutting, and storing them properly keeps them fresh and ready for use in a variety of cuisines.

Adapting recipes:

When it comes to tailoring recipes to particular tastes and dietary limitations, flexibility is essential. The cookbook offers helpful tips for altering dishes to meet the special needs of people with HE, allowing them to enjoy tasty meals without jeopardizing their health.

Suggestions for recipe adaptations include replacing allergenic items with suitable substitutes, modifying seasoning to increase flavor without using too much salt or sugar, and experimenting with different cooking methods to optimize nutrient retention and flavor profile. Individuals can personalize their culinary experience while staying on track with their nutritional objectives by promoting creativity and experimentation in the kitchen.

CHAPTER EIGHT

The Hashimoto's Encephalopathy (HE) Management Diet Cookbook dedicates a full chapter, Chapter 8, to typical concerns and often asked issues about dietary management. This chapter provides a complete guide to navigating the numerous problems that individuals may have when following the recommended dietary program for controlling Hashimoto's Encephalopathy.

Addressing dietary challenges:

One of the most typical challenges people have when following a specialized diet for HE is dealing with cravings and managing social situations. Cravings for items that may worsen symptoms might be especially difficult to control. The chapter offers techniques to assist people in resisting their cravings, such as including delicious alternatives that follow the nutritional rules.

70

It also provides practical ideas for dealing with social situations, such as packing compliant snacks and discussing dietary needs with hosts ahead of time.

Managing Food intolerances:

Another critical element of HE therapy is detecting and treating food intolerances, which can exacerbate symptoms. The chapter explains how to identify potential trigger foods using exclusion diets or food diaries. It also includes suggestions for replacing problematic items with appropriate substitutes, allowing people to maintain a varied and nutritious diet while reducing symptom flare-ups.

Understanding Medicine Interactions:

Many people with HE may be taking drugs to treat their disease, and it is critical to understand how particular medications interact with dietary choices. The chapter gives thorough information on potential medication interactions as well as practical recommendations on how to change dietary consumption to reduce any negative effects. This includes advice on how to time meals and drugs to maximize absorption and efficacy while minimizing the chance of interactions.

Handling dining out:

Dining out or attending social gatherings might provide particular obstacles for someone on a specialized diet for HE.

To address this worry, the chapter provides helpful tips for understanding menus and making informed dining decisions. It gives advice on how to properly communicate dietary preferences to restaurant staff, as well as suggestions for choosing safe selections that follow established nutritional guidelines. It also explores ways to maintain social relationships while following dietary restrictions, such as organizing meetings at home or recommending non-food-related activities.

Finally, the chapter emphasizes the significance of obtaining additional help and resources for individuals who may want assistance and encouragement as they navigate their HE management path. It recommends credible support networks, internet groups, and healthcare experts with expertise in HE management. The chapter seeks to empower individuals by linking them with useful support networks, allowing them to face the challenges of dietary control with confidence and resilience.

Mindful Eating and Self-Care

Hashimoto's Encephalopathy Management Diet Cookbook emphasizes not only the nutritional side of managing the condition but also the value of mindful eating and self-care. This chapter discusses numerous ways and strategies for improving general well-being through mindful eating and supportive self-care routines.

Developing Mindful Eating Habits

Mindful eating entails being fully present and attentive during meals, savoring each bite, and paying attention to hunger and satiety signals. Here are some strategies to practice mindful eating:

Mindful Awareness: Encourage readers to become more aware of their eating patterns by focusing on the sensations, emotions, and thoughts related to food.

Slow Eating: Advocate for eating at a slower pace so that you may completely experience the flavors, sensations, and acts of nourishing your body.

Engaging the Senses: Encourage readers to use all of their senses while eating, including the colors, scents, tastes, and sounds of their meal.

Gratitude Practice: Incorporate gratitude into mealtime by expressing appreciation for the food and the nourishment it contains.

Prioritizing self-care.

Self-care is essential for controlling Hashimoto's Encephalopathy and maintaining overall health. This section highlights the significance of prioritizing self-care practices:

Physical Self-Care: Encourage readers to prioritize activities that improve physical health, such as regular exercise, enough sleep, and medical checkups.

Emotional Self-Care: Emphasise the need to manage stress, practice self-compassion, and seek help from loved ones or mental health specialists.

Mental Self-Care: Emphasise the value of doing things that engage the mind, such as hobbies, artistic interests, or learning new skills.

Stress-Management Strategies

Stress can increase symptoms of Hashimoto's Encephalopathy, thus stress management practices must be included in daily living.

Offer a variety of relaxation techniques, including deep breathing exercises, meditation, gradual muscular relaxation, and visualization.

Hobbies and Leisure hobbies: Encourage readers to choose hobbies that they like, such as gardening, drawing, listening to music, or spending time in nature, as a method to relax and relieve stress.

Self-Care Rituals: To encourage relaxation and emotional well-being, consider creating self-care rituals such as a relaxing bedtime routine, a morning meditation practice, or frequent pampering sessions.

Finding Balance

Maintaining a healthy diet and lifestyle is critical to long-term success in controlling Hashimoto's Encephalopathy.

Flexible Eating Habits: Emphasise the value of dietary flexibility, allowing for occasional indulgences while remaining committed to overall health goals.

Encourage moderation rather than restriction, supporting a balanced nutritional intake while yet allowing yourself to enjoy your favorite foods in moderation.

Listening to the Body: Encourage readers to listen to their bodies and change their eating patterns based on hunger, fullness, and how various meals make them feel.

Celebrating Progress.

Finally, celebrating accomplishments and milestones on the path to greater health is critical for motivation and morale:

Setting objectives: Encourage readers to develop reasonable and attainable objectives for food, exercise, self-care, and overall health.

Tracking Progress: To stay motivated and engaged, keep track of progress, whether it's symptom improvement, dietary modifications, or personal achievements.

Rewarding Yourself: Encourage readers to reward themselves for achieving milestones, whether with a modest treat, a soothing pastime, or simply acknowledging their efforts and dedication.

Building Healthy Habits: Keeping healthy eating habits and other lifestyle adjustments is critical for long-term success in managing Hashimoto's Encephalopathy. Developing healthy habits entails incorporating long-term practices into one's everyday routine. Here are some strategies to consider.

Gradual modifications: Instead of attempting major overhauls, begin with incremental, attainable modifications to your food and lifestyle. This could include eating more fruits and vegetables, limiting processed meals, or committing to regular exercise in modest increments.

Setting Realistic Goals: Create attainable goals that are consistent with your unique tastes and circumstances. Setting reasonable expectations can reduce frustration and enhance the likelihood of success.

Consistency is essential for developing habits. Try to stick to your healthy eating plan and lifestyle adjustments even during difficult times or when confronted with temptation.

Mindful Eating: Practice awareness when eating by paying attention to hunger and fullness signs and savoring each bite. This can help you avoid overeating and develop a healthier connection with food.

Meal Planning: Plan your meals ahead of time to ensure you have healthful selections on hand. This can help you avoid impulsive food choices and make it easier to stick to your diet plan.

Seeking Variety: Include a wide range of nutrient-dense foods in your diet to ensure that you are reaching your nutritional requirements. Try out fresh recipes and ingredients to keep meals interesting and pleasurable.

Monitoring Progress: Tracking symptoms, food choices, and overall well-being is critical for monitoring progress and making informed changes to your management strategy. Here are several ways to track progress:

Symptom Journaling: Keep a journal to record symptoms including exhaustion, brain fog, mood swings, and any other pertinent ones. Take note of any patterns or triggers that could be affecting your illness.

Food Diary: Keep track of your food choices and how they make you feel. Pay attention to any foods that appear to exacerbate or alleviate your symptoms, and consider making changes accordingly.

Schedule regular check-ins with your healthcare provider to discuss your progress, symptoms, and overall well-being. This can help ensure you're on the right track and receive any necessary adjustments to your management plan.

Adapting to Challenges: Although setbacks and challenges are unavoidable when managing Hashimoto's Encephalopathy, it is critical to remain flexible and adaptable in your approach. Here are some suggestions for overcoming obstacles and adjusting your strategy as needed:

Resilience: Develop resilience to overcome setbacks and remain motivated in the face of adversity. Remind yourself that setbacks are a normal part of the trip and provide an opportunity for improvement.

Develop problem-solving skills to deal with challenges as they arise. Instead of perceiving hurdles as impassable barriers, see them as chances to devise novel solutions.

Flexibility: Be willing to change your strategy in response to changing circumstances or new facts. What works for one person may not work for another, so don't be afraid to explore and figure out what works best for you.

Seeking Support: When faced with a dilemma, don't be afraid to seek help from healthcare providers, loved ones, or online groups. Sometimes having someone to lean on can make all the difference in overcoming challenges.

Seeking Continuous Learning: Keeping up with new research, recipes, and tactics for controlling Hashimoto's Encephalopathy is critical for long-term success. Here's how you can engage in continual learning.

.

Experimentation: Be willing to test new recipes, nutritional methods, and lifestyle plans based on fresh research and advice from healthcare professionals.

Embracing a Supportive Community: Connecting with individuals who share similar experiences can provide vital encouragement and support throughout your journey with Hashimoto's Encephalopathy. Here's why joining a supportive community is essential:

Shared Experiences: Talking to people who understand what you're going through can make you feel less alone and more understood. Hearing about other people's experiences and ideas for managing the disease can also provide useful information.

Encouragement: Being a part of a supportive group can give you hope during difficult times and drive you to stick to your management strategy.

 Members of a supportive group may contribute useful advice, recipes, and resources to help you improve your management style and overall well-being.

 Living with a chronic illness such as Hashimoto's Encephalopathy can be emotionally difficult. Having a caring community to turn to for emotional support and understanding can make a big difference in dealing with the ups and downs of the illness.

"Nourishing Neurological Health: Delicious Recipes Packed with Brain-Boosting Ingredients to Support Hashimoto's Encephalopathy Management"

Berry Spinach Smoothie: "Brain Boosting Blend: An Antioxidant-Rich Smoothie with

Berries and Spinach to Support Cognitive Function"

Salmon Salad with Avocado Dressing: "Omega-3 Brain Fuel: Refreshing Salad with Salmon and Creamy Avocado Dressing for Neurological Health"

Subtitle: "Golden Delight: Fragrant Turmeric Coconut Curry with Quinoa for Neuroprotective Benefits"

Broccoli and Cheddar Frittata: "Nutrient-Rich Breakfast: Fluffy Frittata Packed with Broccoli and Cheddar to Nourish the Brain"

Walnut Crusted Chicken Tenders: Title: "Crunchy Goodness: Tender Chicken Tenders Coated with Walnuts for Brain-Boosting Omega-3s"

Spinach and Mushroom Stuffed Bell Peppers: Subtitled "Veggie Powerhouses: Colourful

Bell Peppers Stuffed with Spinach and Mushrooms for Neurological Support"

Sweet Potato and Black Bean Tacos: Subtitled "Plant-Based Fiesta: Flavorful Tacos with Sweet Potatoes and Black Beans to Nourish the Brain"

Title: "Stir-Fry Sensation: Nutrient-Dense Quinoa and Vegetable Medley for Optimal Neurological Function"

Blueberry Almond Overnight Oats: Subtitled "Overnight Indulgence: Creamy Overnight Oats Infused with Blueberries and Almonds for Brain Health"

Crispy Snack Delight: Oven-Roasted Chickpeas Seasoned with Garlic and Rosemary for Cognitive Support"

Sample meal plan:

Week 1:

Day 1:

Breakfast: Blueberry Almond Overnight Oats.

Snack: Berry spinach smoothie.

Lunch: Turmeric Coconut Curry with Quinoa.

Snack: Roasted garlic and rosemary chickpeas.

Dinner: Salmon salad with avocado dressing.

Weeks 2–4:

Maintain a consistent framework, alternating recipes to create variation and prioritize foods that promote brain health.

Prioritise fruits, vegetables, healthy fats, and lean proteins, while limiting processed foods, refined sugars, and artificial additives.

Stay hydrated with water and herbal tea throughout the day.

Prioritise portion control and balanced eating to improve general health and treat symptoms of Hashimoto's Encephalopathy.

THE END

9 7 9 8 3 2 8 0 0 8 8 9 1